The Chadam Protocol

for prevention and treatment of various afflictions using proven safe natural remedies.

Disclaimer: There is no known cure for everything. These processes are recommended from personal use. They have proven effective and safe in overwhelming numbers of cases. I am perfectly well aware that every person reacts in a way determined by their personal DNA, and that what works well for me may not be effective for a given other. No two people have exactly the same DNA chains, not even identical twins. I make no guarantees. I present what evidence and methods have served in my personal experience. When it is information through reports that were not directly in my own experience, I will so state.

Large print. If you need reading glasses or longer arms to read regular print due to the aging process, the Ambrosia section may be able to correct your vision.

Contents

About the author

CD, as he is called now, was born in Florida in 1938. He went to schools through 3 years of college in the area of Tampa, Florida. He later attended universities in other places. His formal education is in botany and genetics. (Spcl. *Orchidacea*)

He worked at his own home from the age of 9 years as a farm worker in a citrus grove and as a counter clerk in a concession stand his parents owned.

His first trip out of the USA was to Honduras, just out of high school. He returned to work in a plant nursery, went to college, and became a hippie in San Francisco, Calif. working for a large orchid grower. While there he joined the musician crowd and played guitar and wrote and arranged music for such as Janis Joplin, *et al.* He traveled over much of the world at that time.

He returned to Florida, where he worked with plant growers and owned a bar. He then moved to Bonita Springs, Florida, and from there to Panamá, where he now makes his residence.

He started writing books in 1983, and has more thn 350 books published at this time (2022) in several genre.

While residing in Panamá he developed a serious cancer, which led to the discovery of the Chadam Protocols.

He now lives in Gualaca, Chiriqui, Panamá, where he does research with native plants, roams the mountains, works with the local Indigenos, plays music with friends, and corresponds with people all over the world through Facebook.

He has a page on FB, <u>Ambrosia peruviana for cancer</u>, where he explains the Chadam Protocol and other medical discoveries. He makes it quite plain he is *not* a medical doctor.

"Chadam" was a company he held with two partners in the USA. He keeps the name because it is also related to his name, <u>CHA</u>rles <u>DA</u>vid <u>M</u>oulton.

I have called for clinical and hospital tests for more than 8 years, even stating that I will supply the basic materials. The only condition is that all information, positive or negative, is dispensed freely. There are no takers, though several wished to try the methods – and were threatened that doing so would result in revocation of their license to practice medicine. I leave it to you to figure who would do such an inhuman thing and why. I have been fighting the big p(harm)s from the first.

Many of the things mentioned here were studied in a ten year study project by the University of Venezuela, and were confirmed. Those studies have about the same chance as a lead butterfly trying to fly over K2 of being accepted by the FDA and AMA – both of which too often seem to be working strictly for the big pharmaceutical companies, not the public.

Be that as it may, I have an open offer to supply the material in the *Ambrosia peruviana* cancer treatment for testing, with the only condition being that all findings, positive or negative, be made public information.

I have enough processed at this writing to treat 50 cases. My area for the growing of the *Amb.*

peruviana and other things, such as curcuma and guava is extremely limited.

I will try to limit this information to what I feel is pertinent to the discovery and preparation of the various items necessary to the protocol. Others may feel certain parts are unnecessary. I will try to avoid bragging or other egocentric tangents, and make it have at least a tenuous connection.

The "About the author" above is more for the fiction works, but expansion of a few points explains how the processes came to be. For example: I was raised on a citrus farm by a large lake in central Florida. Lake Thonotossassa. I was raised with responsibilities from the age of eight.

It was a far different world then. Nothing was thought of my tending a concession stand by myself. If anyone tried to take advantage of the fact I was a little kid, neighbors and passers-by would kick the holy living hell out of them, as was demonstrated twice between the ages of 8 and 10.

The pertinent part is that there are native orchids, such as *Epidendrum tampense* (Now *Encyclia tampensis*), *Epidendrum conopseum, Eulophia alta,* and several other species that led to my interest in botany, with the orchids always of special interest.

An aside: In my science fiction series, *Flight of the Maita*, many stories are based on what little insignificant seeming things can do to influence the future of a person, race, world, or even a galactic society in a few years or thousands of years. Exploring realities and possibilities led to such tales as *Us Barbarians*, where introducing script and calenders in an age of barbaric pirates and such could change the future of the world from violence, wars, and mistrust to a cooperative society.

What little almost unnoticed thing changed a direction in *your* life? A single harsh or an understanding word can change the entire direction of a life. A touch, or a rejection can fix a mental state. History is made by a combination of timing and minutiae. A poet changed an impression we were brainwashed into from birth in my lifetime *(Blowin' in the Wind* – Dylan) and the war-for-profit idea (*Ruby* – Tillis).

They slapped us in the face with the disgusting realities of what we had become.

True; it was deteriorated, deliberately, later, but the basic ideas were brought to the forefront, and will change the direction, politically, later. That is societal evolution. We are living at a time when the barbarians are no longer at the gate, they are occupying and controlling the city. We have the ability to change the direction from stagnation back to dynamism – but will we?

Soapboxing, but there is a point. The pendulum has now swung to the other end, but the lessons are there if we will only realize them. We can either move on in evolving, or we can stagnate. Stagnation is extinction. A few will possibly survive, but will they take the direction of permanent stagnation, like the alligator, or of dynamism, like the birds?

Little things have huge influences in future situations. I went to high school with a friend, Robert Whitman. His brother was Slim Whitman. Slim taught me a few chords on a guitar. That led, several years later, to my being a studio guitarist with Janis Joplin, et al, and my traveling over much of the world, as those native orchids led me to other places and to San Francisco, where the guitar bit placed me into the hippie music scene.

There was much more to the hippie era that was an influence in my personal life and approach to personal relationships that are not pertinent here. I will only say it expanded my sex addiction, and made me see, *before* any experimentation, that the drug scene was a long road to nowhere, and that the propaganda we were being fed was mostly BS. Overall, it was negative.

I do not class marijuana with most other drugs. It is less debilitating than alcohol or nicotine. It has some tremen-dous medical advantages. Like most such things, no two people react the same to anything. It is a matter of how it affects *you*. Cocaine, while it has little affect to me, can destroy others. To some, it is quite useful, to others, it is damaging. It is also a matter of processing. Crack is not good to any I have ever known who used it. Opiates have extensive positive properties to medicine for many, but leads to Hell for others. This is true of most drugs.

So! Back to where this was supposedly heading!

The point of the diatribe is that a little thing can have huge effect on the future, and we can't know, at the time, what they portend.

In high school, in Vo-Ag, Everyone had cows and pigs and chickens and, in one case, goats.

I had orchids. That made me the butt of many jokes. I must be gay! (It was "queer" back then.)

Then came the proms. All the others could give their dates a rose or a carnation. I could give my date a dozen orchids. Then, a carnation was 25 cents, a rose as much as 50 cents. Orchid corsages started at $5.00. I gave Lavonne both a corsage orchid and a wrist corsage archid! I gave her mother a stem of 14 *C. bowringeana* orchids to put on the kitchen table! That was $28 value. Today, that would be giving her $450 to sit on the kitchen table!

Guess who had ten of the most popular girls vying for being his date!

I already had a bit of a reputation as being expert on orchids. All the rest of the guys had jobs in stores, carrying groceries or stocking shelves. I had a trip, all expenses paid, to Honduras to gather and classify orchids for an advertising agency. It was the era of the orchid wars, where people would even kill to have a new orchid discovered and named after them. After all, Col. Cattley was world renowned, and he only named an orchid he bloomed from a shipment from Colombia! Today, the Cattleya and its hybrids are a great part of the cut flower trade, as well as a major part of the collectors' plants. There are millions of collectors and casual orchid growers in just the USA.

That led to other expense paid trips, and huge changes in my personal life. On one such trip, when I stayed in Honduras for more than a year, I met a voodoo papaloi. I never believed in that crap, but I saw and experienced some things that were and are unexplainable by anything observed then or since.

That led to an experience in Florida that I wrote about that has never been explained, but that seemed to answer a few questions. (*The von Artle Legacy*). It amounted to a ghost story. I don't believe in ghosts, but something very weird was going on there. "Tom" gave an explanation of hauntings of the type claimed in those old castles that made some sense.

Ever get one of those cards that have a small silicon crystal that plays a song or message when you open the card? Modern computers are run by much the same process.

Those old castles are built of granite. Granite contains a bunch of small crystals ...

He also explained exorcisms could work under

specific conditions. Remember that it takes a millivolt to program or erase the crystal, and many people can produce a "psychic" millivolt.

A very small thing can produce an enormous response. According to the Zero Theory, it can even produce an omniverse.

Then a few years back, in Florida, where I formed a company, Spectrascape, with a partner whose father owned a small beer and wine bar. We did some larger landscape jobs in an upscale community. The place I was living was across the street from an auto salvage (junkyard) operation. I was always good at auto mechanics (though I did *not* like it) and worked there some while, due to an inlaw lawyer with a firm partner politician, getting a full liquor license for the beer bar. We became the top live rock bar in the area.

There was a nudist camp nearby, and it was to be a joke when I was invited there by a resident. Either I was to be shocked and refuse to go, or was to go and be embarrassed. Great fun!

Well, I had been a musician in San Francisco and all over much of the world – that they did not know. I was perfectly comfortable in a nude group. I was also a sex addict, which a few of them knew, so it was a joke that backfired.

I met a woman who was a so-called expert on natural medicines. She pointed out that major medical break-throughs were mostly recognizing old folk remedies worked. Digitalis, which I had growing in my own garden. Penicillin, which was bread mold, etc.

I understood that there was some potential there, but most of it was hype and BS, in my estimation. An easy way for charlatans to scam people out of a few bucks.

I moved from there to Bonita Springs. I had already written several books, and even had a couple considered for publishing by the trads. I had an Atari computer and a dot matrix printer, Epson, which was the top of the line – but editors would not accept less than a laser-printed MS.

Bummer!

Then Lulu. I gave the trads, even the one who had printed a work (That sold exactly $137.22 more than the advance), the finger. I started the POD route. I was making good returns for the work, and became a fairly large part of the original establishing of the site and POD printing.

Then the yuppies took over Lulu and the volume-over-quality fixation took over POD publishing. An idea with huge potential for quality work was suddenly just another way to make millions with no effort and no ethics. I had been with Lulu since the inception, more than 25 years, and was being treated like a new teenage no-talent amateur mark.

In other words, they sold out, just as predicted. Now it was all silly romances written by teenage girls and sillier adventures written by teenage boys just to be able to say they wrote a book. The time when you could have a "best-seller" by offering it free on the eBook market, such as Amazon or Smashwords, was upon us. Serious writers were now in competition with the freebies. Thousands of new titles per week. Maybe two were worth that price.

The deterioration of the mediums has continued, steadily gaining momentum. Special interests have garnered con-trol of them, and can stop distribution of works (such as this) through funding-control. "If you print that one, all advertising and research funding from Garbage Bag Pharmaceuticals will cease. Immediately!"

In other words, it is lobbying the same as with congress and other politicians. Threats and bribes. It is how business is today.

Another soapbox. Maybe enough to reach the page limits.

Things rocked along dully in Bonita Springs. I wrote the CD Grimes, PI, Det. Lt. Nick Storie Mysteries, and the Flight of the Maita series, and a lot of other things.

I had an encounter with folk medicine then, that directed my ideas to a more liberal view of folk medicines.

A local boy was swimming in a stillwater pond, and became infected with an amoeba that attacks the brain. The subject develops high fever, goes into a coma, and dies. Always.

I had come across an affliction in Malaysia called "Brain fever." It was caused by swimming in stillwater ponds. It was regularly cured with a decoction made from an orchid, *Dendrobium cruminatum*, which was the only reason I ever heard of it.

I had a plant in my own greenhouse.

I contacted the hospital where the boy died. I was passed to a doctor who was in charge of that kind of disease.

He first asked what my medical degree was.

I said my education was in botany and genetics. I had no medical degree.

Then I wasn't "qualified" to make suggestions to the lofty royal super-educated megabrain doctors in charge of research concerning such infections – was I?

I was dismissed. No further contact, no even listening to what I had to say. After all, if there were such a cure, the big pharms would have researched it and produced a concentrate for their use – wouldn't they?

I can't know for certain if it is the same infection. If it is, how many have died because research on a *non-patentable* cure was never done (– was it?)

My mother died, at 102 years, and I came to Panamá at the suggestion of a friend (of sorts) in music, who was into the Save the Manatees bit. He said I would never go back to Florida. Bocas del Toro was the perfect fit with my personality.

He was right. I went back to Florida to sell my property and get out! The politics in Florida were disgusting and corrupt, and getting (and have gotten) steadily worse.

I had a lot of cash from the sale of my property at the peak of the market. Very soon after my move, the bottom fell out. The final balloon payment was forgiven, as repossession would result in a taxation that exceeded the resulting value of the property (From $800K+ to, *because* of those taxes, $0.00)

I was subsequently scammed out of my entire retirement, but that is pertinent here only because it led to the later situation. (Free eBook: *Fading Paradise*)

I really didn't much care about the loss of the property and funds, personally. It bothered me because my partner lost his part he was going to leave to his daughters. He later went back to California, invented a device, was going to receive several million dollars, and was (in my belief) murdered for it. I could present a fairly concise case for investigation, such as the invention and agreements were never even revealed to his daughters, but that would go the way the "investigation" (refused) by the fiscalia here in Panamá went. There is even more corruption in the states than here, but it is not as blatant, thus is not perceived by far too much of the public.

I was in telephone contact with Kevin, weekly, and knew about the invention and other things he was planning. The daughters were never told of the invention and patent. The patent lawyer was at the party where Kevin had the "freak accident" that killed him. The party was to celebrate the contract where he was to be paid two hundred thousand dollars immediately, with a minimum guarantee of two million dollars within two years. Kevin told me about it the day before when he called me to do exactly that, and to say he was filling a container with things, such as guitars and amplifiers to replace the Gibson SG I gave him to finance his going to California.

He had not told his daughters about the invention, because he was intending to surprise them with it when they resolved a couple of problems with a sister or sister-in-law who had caused a rift between him and one daughter.

I have this wonderful lot for sale very cheap! It has a beautiful view of a lush valley on one side and a view of the sewage plant on the other. I will sell it to you at a huge discount! Only to you, though. Don't tell anyone else about it!

That's too obvious for a scenario in one of my murder mysteries. There *is* no mystery, IMO. Only an honest investigation would determine if my opinion is correct. That will not happen.

Things went along. I was involved in the orchid research, spent a lot of time in the mountains, played music in local bars, and wrote many of the Clint Faraday Mysteries. I was collecting aluminum while in the mountains for extra money and to pay for the trips. Life was rather pleasant. I was borderline broke from giving whatever I had to friends who were experiencing hard times, but didn't care.

A friend in David developed a lymphoma, tried a lot of the scam cures, and died from it. I later learned that the procedures, which were just money drains, in his case, had preventive value, but not cure value.

They did have that preventive value, and some symp-tomatic relief value. They were not as useless as I had thought.

Then I developed a lymphoma. It was growing rapidly. It would cost me over $4000 in the hospitals here (probably $85K in the states), and under contract where I would have to take the chemo and radiation – which were already shown as of little or even negative effectiveness.

I couldn't come up with $400, at the time, much less $4K.

I saw a post on Facebook, shared by Ken McFadden, that said a plant, *Artemisia annua*, could cure cancer cheaply and quickly. It was known since 1976, when the critical ferrotopsis catalyst was discovered.

I researched *Art. Annua*. I, a botanist, noted that a plant of it was growing right outside my kitchen door!

(The reason I mentioned I am a botanist is

because I misidentified *Ambrosia peruviana* as *Art. annua*. My defense is that *Amb. peruviana* is synonymous with *Amb. artimisiafolia*, and the different in description of the species is mostly that the seeds of *Art. annua* are small and dustlike, while *Amb. peruviana* has small nodular hard seeds. Also, *Art. annua* is not found in Panamá, while *Art. absinthe*, which is of rather limited use for cancer, is.)

I immediately intensively researched *Art. annua* to determine use, restrictions, contra-indications, and any-thing else known of its use. I found that there were few dangers, that certain things were critical to use, that it was safer than most extant medications. The optimum use was averaged, and I tried it.

That original dosage and ingestion is the same as the protocol now, with little change. By pure luck, I seem to have stumbled upon the more effective way to utilize the information gathered. It was also by accident the *Amb. peruviana* was discovered to be the actual plant in use.

It worked!

I started the first dose, after the iron tablet was taken at 4:00 AM, at 7:30 AM. The second dose was at 11:30 AM. The constant itching was far less, and the inflammation was reduced to almost none. The third dose was at 3:30 PM. The itching was gone, and the oozing was almost gone. The inflammation was gone. The final dose was at 7:30

PM. The knot was still there, but was only ... there. There was no itching, oozing, or inflammation. I could touch it, and there was no pain.

The following day, there were no symptoms, except the knot. It was dry.

Three days later, it was noticeably smaller.

I had purchased the dried Altamisa I still thought was Artemisia in a local herbalist shop. I found a vendor near the hospital that has some fresh plant for sale, so bought it all.

At that time, I had exactly $6.49 invested – and had relieved all symptoms, if not cured, a stage 4 lymphoma!

I decided my research was only beginning. A friend who runs a pensión had a man staying in the pensión who had liver cancer, complicated with cirrhosis, that his doctors said would kill him within 4 days. He had been following my use, so said there was nothing to lose, so as much as force-fed the protocol to him. He was in a semi-coma, and wasn't much aware of any of it.

The following day, he was aware and able to move about a bit.

The next, he got out of bed and went to the baño. In the afternoon, he went to the porch to sit and talk.

The next, he was able to walk around town.

His doctors could not explain why the cancer was, seemingly, arrested, even dead. The cirrhosis was also greatly relieved!

Two weeks later, he went back to Germany. No cancer, no serious cirrhosis.

The man, Lee Hare, and his son, Bret, started an intense study of the plant. His son quickly discovered that *Art. annua* didn't grow in Panamá, but that *Amb. peruviana* did, and it was even described as being synonymous with *Amb. artimisiafolia*, which name suggests the plants look the same. I then discovered the seed difference in the species, and the structures that produced those seeds was different.

We then tested the protocol with total success. It seemed to be more effective against certain forms of cancer than *Art. annua*. It cured breast cancer and all mets very quickly and completely, as well as lung cancer, prostate cancer (in my own case! It appears the lymphoma was a met from prostate cancer I was unaware of.) The only cancers we have experience with that are slow to respond are certain skin cancers.

We have since discovered bewares, such as oils, and positive side-effects, such as reinvigoration of eyesight lost to problems due to the aging process in many.

This led me from the belief that natural cures were BS and scams, to the greatest degree, to the knowledge that *some* of them are real and effective, even where chemical and such as radiation treatment are not.

As an example; I had chronic arthritis for years

before moving here to Panamá. Just moving here relieved it to a great extent, but I was limited in movement and in pain when a weather front moved through, or such.

The Indio woman who suggested a possible relief from the cancer with "Altimisa, that plant right there," said guava leaf tea would take care of those kinds of body pains. Another thing that worked far better than even hoped for. That was eight years ago last February 15 (The day after Valentine's Day is why I remember it). I have not had any pain, except for a slight nagging when a severe front (that caused an innundation) passed through.

It is also a sleep aid and mood enhancer.

My research also led to other cures/treatments that seem to be effective for many. *i.e.* Cinnamon (*real* cinnamon, not cassia, which is what is sold for flavoring in most places as cinnamon) relieves any fungus problem, as well as other things, such as high blood pressure.

Other things will be described in the text. Such as how Coconut oil can cleanse the veins and arteries and remove clots. It can even make hair grow back after loss to male pattern balding.

There are a number of things that will not be included here. Plants of the Calendula group are very good for upset stomach and such.

Valerian is a good sleep enhancer.

Cannabis is not among the things included, mostly because it is so wide-spectrum, and has been and is being exhaustively researched by others

Ginger is a very good remedy for relief from motion sickness and seasickness.

There are hundreds of such things, and my time is too limited to try to study them all.

Cinnamomum verum NOT *Cinnamomum cassia*

Cinnamomum cassia is generally sold in stores for flavoring. It is not effective for fungus control. I am told that real cinnamon can be purchased as Ceylon Cinnamon.

I have used cinnamon for the cure of toenail fungus, and in orchids for supposedly incurable fungi, with success.

For toenail fungus, sprinkle cinnamon powder into a sock and wear it for several hours. It is uncomfortable, but not painful.

<u>I am told by usually credible sources</u>: For yeast bloom and other intestinal outbreaks, a teaspoon of cinnamon in warm water as a tea. The reports are that it is effective in all internal fungal infections, such as in vaginal outbreaks.

<u>I am told by usually credible sources</u>: cinnamon tea can reduce blood pressure with continued used over a period of time.

<u>I am told by usually credible sources</u>: cinnamon used as a tea can control blood sugar levels and greatly aid against diabetes.

Again, this is with "real" cinnamon, not *C. cassia*

Azadiracha indica

Neem: China Berry

<u>I am told by usually credible sources</u>: Neem oil is the only effective treatment against psoriasis. There is much variation in how to use and dosage for me to suggest anything. I have read two websites that claim it can be a cure, which I tend to doubt, as it is a genetic affliction, and that it can render complete symptomatic relief, which I can accept as not unlikely.

I have done little research, as my time is too limited. There are other claims, but I feel, as this is the only sug-gested relief for psoriasis that is credible, it should be included here.

Coffees in today's markets are mostly varieties of *C. arabica* that are hybridized for growing in specific places. The flavor variations are partly due to soils and altitudes.

Before taking coffee in any quantity, one must determine personal genetic traits that are not debilitating. Coffee contains such ingredients as caffeine, which are of various effects to various individuals. I have consumed an average of 8 cups per day for 35 years. No detectable ill effects. My ladyfriend gets hyper with 1 cup

This is included because of my own *annectdotal* report. With consideration of a long term study by a German panel that determined that *long-term* ingestion of a minimum of 4 cups per day generally results in no Alzheimer's mental aberrations. The suggestion seems to be that long-term use of the beverage purges/prevents aluminum build-up in the brain.

This in turn suggests that, if you are under, say, 25 years of age and start the daily ingestion, you will not develop Alzheimer's in later life, but if you are already past, say, 50 years of age, it is unlikely it will significantly help.

Again: determine first if you will react positively to this extreme, seeming, protocol.

Family history also figures into it. If your family

is prone to Alzheimer's, you should perhaps investigate the method.

This is another where I have extensive personal experience using. It has a lot of uses that are generally unknown, is available in the tropicals and much of the temperate zones.

The fruits are of some use to pregnant women for various minerals, vitamins, and other ingredients, but are not the main reason for inclusion here.

The leaves are amazing in their uses.

My first exposure to the medicinal uses were at the time of the *Ambrosia peruviana* cancer cure discovery. I came across an article that claimed the extract from the leaves is a definite way to prevent hangovers from excess alcoholic beverage consumption. It was for a commercial product.

Well, I was not prone to hangovers to any extent. I always enjoyed a few beers and conversation or when playing guitar in local establishments. I would sometimes have a few tequilas, which never gave me a hangover, or some rum, which did. There was a note that it stopped pain from sciatica.

That got a response! I had a couple of sciatica attacks in the not-distant past!

I was working on the protocol for cancer. There was a large guava tree next to the carport where I was staying at the time. I was in the kitchen anyhow, so made up a bit of the extract to have on hand when/if I needed it. That was on a Friday, and I was going to be in David with friends to jam and play some guitar in a local bar. I had performed before with these same talented people, and enjoyed the time immensely – but they tended to drink a bit too much rum.

I had a bottle of the extract in my maleta, everything was tranquilo, we would probably drink a lot. It would start with beer and segue into rum.

I would deliberately drink too much. Why not? I could see if the guava leaf extract worked to specifications!

Besides; my arthritis was bothering me, and that, at least, would be lessened with the rum, though beer also helped.

To make it shorter, I drank a good bit more than I had planned. I was slurring my words and even staggering a bit. I finally realized I was overdoing it, and said my good nights and went back to the pensión, if rather unsteadily. I managed to slam my shoulder into the jamb on the gate, and it was hurting like Hell.

I talked to a couple of people on the porch, and one of them suggested, rather pointedly, that I should go to bed.

I went to my room and took a slug of the extract, then did the teeth washing and such.

I remember that it was twenty minutes since I took the extract. I suddenly didn't have any pain from the bruised shoulder, and the arthritis pain was gone! My thinking was back to normal! I said a tongue-twisting phrase, Big Black Bug's Blood, and didn't slur it!

I put on a shirt and pants and went back out front. I saw Tom roll his eyes.

I still staggered a bit, if not nearly as much, but could speak and think clearly. They didn't believe it!

I still had a buzz, but it wasn't affecting my thoughts or voice. The body pains were gone!

Soon, it was to bed. Sleep was deep and resting. No hint of a hangover.

The next day, I was starting to get the arthritis pains again, if less. I drank a shot glass of the extract. In twenty minutes, the pain was gone. I could bend and twist like I hadn't been able to in years, it seemed!

I couldn't help but notice I was in a better mood than for some time, too. I put that to the fact the pain was gone.

A week working with the *Amb. peruviana*, then back to David. I had determined that taking a dose every 8 hours kept me pain free. My mood was very up all the time.

This time, I took a bit (I had determined about 3/4 of a shot was good for 8 hours) before I went to the bar. I drank much like the week before.

I did not get drunk. I got a pleasant buzz. I noted that there were some physical effects, but no detrimental mental effects.

I had slept well since that first night. My mood stayed high. I had no body pains.

There were several people in the bar across from my house that tended to drink too much, and had hangovers. I took the, what I was calling No Goma (No Hangover) to the bar, and everyone tried it. Nobody got belligerent, nobody had a hangover the next day.

I started selling a half pint rum bottle of the extract for a dollar and a half. Everybody was buying it.

Then I told them how to make their own. A lot of people have a guava tree in their yard here, or there is one close, growing by the roadside. My market disappeared overnight.

C'est la vie!

(A national sort of joke: a Frenchman and a Latino were in a cantina. They could just barely communicate when a beautiful girl in the traditional flowing skirt came to lean over the bar, talking to the bartender. The door opened, and a sudden gust blew the skirt up. She didn't have a stitch on underneath. The Frenchman said, typically, "C'est la vie!" The Latino replied, "Yo tambien!"

Phonetically, c'est la vie – that is life – is the same as the Spanish, se la vie - I saw it.)

Back to reality.

I had an idea! No! Really!

A town drunk came in to cadge a few shots of

rum from the customers. I talked him into trying the extract Ken kept behind the bar. He said he felt better than he could remember feeling after about twenty minutes (We since determined that was the time the effects of the extract "Kicked in.") I gave him a bottle. He soon said, in effect, "I am a real pain in the ass, aren't I?"

Three nights later, he was in the bar, having a beer. We talked, and he said he had to go to a job interview. He left almost a half bottle of beer on the counter!

He has since gotten a job and cleaned himself up. He drinks a beer or two, or has a shot, but walks away from more. He has a guava tree, or his next-door neighbor does, and makes his own extract.

I don't know if it will have the same effect on other alcoholics, but think it is a thing that must be researched.

Another *unconfirmed* claim is that regular use can cause hair loss can be prevented, even reversed, by use of the extract. I must note that my own hairline was rapidly receding when I first used it, and has not receded more since. This may be a result of the Ambrosia or of the guava or the combination. Another place where more research is needed.

For cosmetic purposes, some amazing results can be shown by certain uses. They are temporary, to a great extent. I am, if the time is found, trying to find a way to stabilize the results. This is one thing, as it is a vanity issue, I will reserve for a time when it will produce a profit. After all, the rest of this has been at personal expense to me to discover, use, and give away.

Guava: <u>*The Preparation*</u>

We have determined that the shelf life of the dried leaves is in excess of one year.

Take the older leaves. Not the newest three or four. It appears that those grown at altitude are marginally stronger than the ones from lower elevations. The processing makes that a "no difference" statement.

You may use the leaves immediately, or dry them for later use. Simply put the leaves in a dry place until they are obviously desicated enough for storage. That can be as little as forty eight hours.

The preparation of the extract is quite simple. You simply put about 3 larger leaves per each two cups of water and boil until a white residue begins to form. We use ½ pint rum bottles, sterilize them with Clorox or equivalent, 1 part to twenty parts water. Include caps in the sterilization. Drain, and replace the caps. Remove the caps only long enough to pour in the *hot* extract, and reseal.

Place the bottles of extract in a low-light area. They can be stored for eight months or more with no lessening of effect.

The only contamination we have found is an occasional growth of aspergillus fungus. Some people are highly allergic to aspergillus. It floats on top as a blob of slime. It may be strained out, the extract brought to a boil, and used. We strain through a coffee sock.

Guava leaf extract has a number of uses. Topical uses are as a skin replenisher or as a reliever from insect bites. It is excellent as a relief of minor and more serious irritations, such as the skin parasites I have that have no known cure. Relief is both from the protocol and topical application.

Itching or red eyes are relieved quickly and completely. It may be sprayer/dropped directly into the eyes.

I have been told by usually reliable sources: it does not have the same side-effects as Visine etc. and can be used against pink-eye. This needs further investigation. Use with extreme caution.

It can amaze you how it clears the complexion. It aids in healing may sores and cuts.

I keep a spray bottle of the extract ready at all times.

For internal relieving of many things, as well as the no hangover, the pain relief (arthritis, sciatica, joint and muscle pains. Migraines, and other body pains) the protocol is effective.

It is a sleep aid. This is, as with other uses, timed at about twenty minutes before going to bed. You sleep soundly and restfully.

It is a starch blocker. It stops starches in the diet from converting into sugars, allowing the food to pass through the system without being absorbed into the bloodstream. This can be a tremendous aid to diabetics. After a meal containing the starches in many foods (Rice, potatoes, pasta, and other basic foods), take a dose, and blood sugars remain stable and low.

It can aid in diets to lose weight, in that excess sugars are no longer a basic factor. It is not for weight loss, but is for no weight gain.

I have been told by usually reliable sources: longer term usage lowers and stabilizes blood pressure.

My personal experience is that I had high/normal blood pressure that would spike dangerously at times. I paid little attention to that fact, as it was never a problem here in Panamá. While it was high/normal, it no longer spiked.

I has a ministroke recently (that was borderline a full stroke) when my neighbor came in to aid me. I lost all sense of balance. And couldn't walk across the room without falling on my face. His wife called an ambulance. A doctora and two nurses came. They gave me every test they had available. Everything was great for a person twenty years younger. My brain waves were stable, as was everything else. _My blood pressure was low/normal_ and stable.

I cannot say it was the guava leaf extract or the _Ambrosia peruviana_ – or the combination. It requires investigation.

I am in Panamá, and am over the age of 75. What

would have cost me more than three thousand eight hundred dollars in the more liberal states in the USA cost me $0.00. Of course, Panamá cares about its citizens and visitors.

Mosquito repellant. I find that, when in the presence of people who are being bitten by mosquitos, I am not. Occasionally, I will receive one bite, usually around the ankles, in a place where there are a lot of mosquitos.

Again, this could be guava or Amb. or both.

It has cosmetic uses.

<u>*The protocol*</u>

2/3 liquid ounce of extract by mouth every 6-8 hours.

That's it. In the eight years I have used it, the time between doses has lessened only two hours. I sometimes don't use it for twenty four hours. It seems to repair the damage that results in arthritis. A friend has had excellent results treating rotator cup damage. That needs further research.

I have no personal experience with migraines. Several people have reported it works. A study says it is effective on about 65% of subjects tested. The same study says it is effective in slightly more cases of sciatica.

<u>Ambrosia peruviana</u>:
Altamis(a) Western Ragweed, *et al*

I make no claims, other than what is presented here is true in my personal experience. I do *not* claim it will work in every case. The protocol needs clinical/hospital testing.

That testing is refused every time it is proposed for more than 8 years. The few who would do the research/testing were threatened with loss of their license to practice medicine. I have been threatened, personally, but in a way I could not prove it against an individual, organization, or for profit business. I have no doubt whatever where the threats came from, because I asked who or what could profit from the information being blocked from widespread know-ledge of the data.

Combine that with the facty that cancer treatment is a, I am told, $310B/yr. *business*, and the answer becomes all too obvious. I am being threatened by egregious greedbags if I disburse information that may negatively impact their profit margin. It is to the point where printing of a book that holds that information is blocked from print, even eBook distribution.

I am aware that the distributors are within their rights to refuse anything at their discretion.

I am also aware that there are numerous scams

extant that prey on the fears of people through scams and sometimes outright misinformation. I find much of the negative "disinformation" is produced and placed by those same entities that wish to stop the availability of true information.

I also believe that the information and/or scams should be required of proof if presented, which would remove most of the scams from the market. Expose the charlatans as being what they are. Presenting a half-truth is the most effective lie. Stating that massive dosage of vitamin"C" can be a preventative is certifiable truth. That it is a cure is a deliberate lie. Charlatans can garner huge profits with that scam – and, in my opinion, kill people.

This can be handled through a few tests. Using the word "Cure" in a title should not be a basis for censorship when the author can produce multiple witnesses on which the process has succeeded.

The amount of profit must be considered. If a book is to be an advertisement for a business, such information should be required on the cover. It is a simple solution, and could be like the FB notation on a meme/post: "Sponsored."

I have, in all my books on the subject, stated that there are no claims made about the effectiveness of whatever. No promises, and specifically mention of the fact that no one thing works the same on all cases. We are different in our genetic makeup in ways that one person's medicine is often another person's poison. That is a fact of reality.

I have, repeatedly, asked for clinical/hospital testing of the protocol. I will provide the materials for the tests. The only conditions are that all information of success or failure becomes public property, immediately. Identification of subjects may, of course, remain purely confidential. Any variations from the protocol must be included in the reports.

The safety of the protocol is established over centuries, even millennia of use. The reports by the study group of the University of Venezuela over ten years shows that the dangers are far less than any of the extant "conventional treatments" used by most hospitals and clinics. It appears that the only contraindication is if there are lesions in the upper digestive tract they may experience extreme discomfort.

Much of the information here is to be found free on the Facebook page: Ambrosia peruviana for cancer.

There are a variety of uses of the plant. Some are vanity uses (though I contend that the improvement in appearance is the result of repairs to the damage to the skin).

It is a necessity of the distributor of a minimum number of pages for a printed book. Were that not a factor, these long diatribes would not be included in the book. I will try to make them somehow connected to the thrust, and tend to get political. I apologize for any excesses.

Asthma
Cancer
Cirrhosis
Complexion
Constipation/diarrhea
Hair Growth
HIV
Internal parasites
Leishmaniasis
Liver detox
Lung cleanser
Sleep aid
Virus
Vision

Some of these uses have been shown effective over ten years to study group from University of Venezuela.

The following is mostly taken from the previous three books about the protocol.

This was written with an assumption that I was using *Artemisia annua,* which does not grow here, and is available only through the net. The plant actually used is *Ambrosia peruviana*, a plant called Altamisa here. It has been used for centuries, and is even safer than *Artemisia annua.* I'm a botanist, and was in too much of a hurry to go through the entire data. It looks, smells, and tastes like *Artemisia annua*, and is proven safe, so I used it. A friend pointed out that it was different, though very closely similar. The basic visible difference is that *Artemisia* has tiny powdery seeds, while *Ambrosia* has small globular seeds.

In editing this, I tried to change the names everywhere it appeared. The use is identical, and the *Ambrosia* appears to be even more wide spectrum. Discoveries in January of this year (2019) indicate it is found in all the Americas, and has been introduced to Europe and Asia during WWI. It is generally considered an invasive, noxious weed.

Who'd'a thought!

Cautionary note for those using the Ambrosia peruviana treatment for cancer: I recently posted that we are using coconut oil as a carrier, as an experiment.

It is *negative* in effect. Do *not* use oils as a carrier.

Use fats, such as butterfat [the reason I stress *whole* milk], or the fat that floats out when you prepare chicken stock/soup. [For the soup, I cool the stock, and the fat solidifies on top, where it is easily skimmed off. I then add a teaspoon of the fat to clear stock per cup, and use it as herein suggested for use with milk. Heat it *slightly*, to where the fat is liquid. Do *not* overheat, as that destroys some of the critical ingredients]. The chicken fat hides the bad taste of the Ambrosia quite well.

This is the reason I stress: DO NOT MIX PROTOCOLS, as one can nullify another.

If you add something, or use mixed methods, and it fails, please do not claim that my protocol failed. *Yours* did.

If you try additions or mixes and they fail or work, I would appreciate the information, as it adds to the data collection process.

There was a small note on a website that deals with medicinal plant research that claimed a group had discovered that a plant used in medicine for more than two thousand years had been proven more than some-odd thousand times more effective than chemotherapy following cancer operations. It was claimed that it was far more effective than guanabana.

I had a cancer on my forehead that was just lately beginning to grow rapidly and cause discomfort with itching and burning sensations. It also bled, at times.

A friend, Chris Mullener, had recently died from much the same kind of cancer. He had refused standard chemotherapy, and was spending his entire life's savings seeking cures from obvious charlatans, such as massive vitamin C and Black Salve treatments.

My problem was that I am in Panamá, where Medicare etc. is not available. I am living on minimum Social Security, plus a small amount of royalties. I could not begin to afford treatment, much less surgery.

I immediately researched as much as was available on the net having to do with the herb. There is extensive material from the WHO to hundreds of blogs and medical research sites.

I rejected the more extravagant claims and those about studies by the big drug companies. The more extreme positive sites were people who had an experience where it seemed like a miracle cure for a number of things.

It had been proven to stop malaria, though with reappearance of the symptoms after a short while, in many cases. It does stop the disease for long enough to get proper treatment. (I wonder if it will also stop dengue, a very serious problem here). It cures Leishmaniasis (as does Praziquantel, which is not available here, where it is most needed, and ivermectin [not confirmed]). The drug companies have their own products, based on antimony, which are expensive and dangerous, in some cases.

A friend's young son recently died of visceral Leishmaniasis. The treatment is not recommended for children less than six years old. The boy was four. He reacted to the antimony. Nothing else was tried. I feel the blood of that boy and countless others are on the hands of the doctors who give a treatment counter-recommended, and the drug companies, who do not allow Praziquantel to be prescribed here.

The drug companies put out a lot of false information supplied by special "Scientific medical researchers" about anything that will cut into their profit margins. Twenty cents worth of antimony compounds are sold for more than $400 for the cure in use and misuse.

The preparation for the natural tea that can cure Leishmaniasis and other things was "tested" by the drug company, and found worthless.

Reading their test preparations and results made it obvious why it failed. They used one third of the recommended dosage, and boiled it, which is known to destroy the active ingredients. These were the same "scientific researchers" who found that tobacco did not adversely affect health in the 1960's.

Yeah, unh-hunh, sure, and right!

I came across a paper that stated that, by adding an iron supplement tablet to the treatment, prostate cancer was cured in very short time. It only mentioned prostate cancer with a short note that it appeared to lessen or cure colon cancer.

I have an enlarged prostate that caused a lot of discomfort, particularly difficulty and frequency of urination. A single beer before going to bed meant getting up at least three times per night.

I have had no tests, but felt that I was a candidate for prostate cancer. I'm 76, and am in the very high risk group. My father died of cancer that started in the prostate and spread to the kidneys and bones.

The herb is readily available here. The herbalists sell it dried. The research showed it is effective for several months, if properly dried and stored, despite the drug companies claiming it was subject to mold, which it is not, and rapid deterioration, which it is not, if handled with a small amount of care, mainly not allowing it to get damp and too warm at the same time.

I have a small plant right outside the kitchen door, though it is much too small to produce the dosage necessary.

I was walking by a herbalist in a nearby city and decided to ask. Nothing ventured, nothing gained (how trite!).

Oh, yes! They had it! $3.60 for enough for the recommended dosage.

So I bought enough for two treatments. I stopped by a farmacia on the way back to the bus and bought some iron supplement tablets ($0.65). I had a blender. I bought a liter of whole milk ($1.76).

I would have personal evidence, pro or con, in a couple of weeks. It was damned well worth a shot!

How I Prepared the Treatment

The plant is *Ambrosia*, called Altamisa in the shops here. There are a number of varieties. *Artemisia annua* was the one mentioned in the cancer cure, which I believed, at the time to be the species here. The active ingredient, artemisinin, is in all of the species. The others have varying amounts of other useful medicines.

I have since learned that *Artemisia annua* does not grow here, that what I was using was *Ambrosia peruviana*, which I will use in the following. The use is the same, in all instances.

The information suggested that the dosage would require 90 grams of the green product, which is about 25 grams dried weight. My two packages of dried leaves and small stems were about 30 grams apiece.

I took an iron tablet. This was about two hours before I took the first dose. One iron tablet is enough for the entire series. You need not take another before each dose.

I picked out the harder stems, put them aside, put the leaves in the blender with the liter of whole milk, liquified the mixture, drank 1/4 of it (tastes truly horrible!) and put the rest in the refrigerator.

On this, I kept shaking it to be able to swallow the ground leaves as well as the milk. The advantage is that the medical products remain in the body much longer, plus you take the entire dosage.

I took the stems, put them in two cups of water, ran the blender to chop them up a bit, put the mixture in a stainless steel pan on the stove (I do not recommend aluminum pans with medicines), brought the temperature to 130 degrees F. *(Do not boil)*, for a few minutes, then strained out the stem pieces and drank 1/4 of that. (Tastes worse than with the milk). [Note: I have since learned that this use was of very little advantage, as the curcumenes and quercetin are of very low solubility in water. The milk contains butterfat, which is an excellent carrier, and easily absorbed by the body. I now do the same with the stems, but use whole milk instead of water. It appears to work quite well, though I would hesitate to make it the whole process.]

I took the rest of it in 3 more doses 4 hours apart.

Now to wait a couple of weeks to see if it really works!

I usually have a couple of beers before going to bed, more because I talk with friends then than because of the beer, though it makes me sleep a bit more. I never sleep more than five hours a night. Four with no beer, as much as six with too many beers, though the more beer, the more wake-ups for urination.

I had about two hours when I felt slightly dizzy, but no other side effects I noticed.

The nest day was a normal type day. I had the two beers, as was my routine. There was no itching or burning from the cancer or from the parasites (cystocercosis ?) I'm fighting. The lesions from the parasites were far less inflamed.

Right on! There was that, if nothing else. It was already worth it for a day of feeling normal!

Next day was even better. I had about six beers that night, as we watched the game on TV and celebrated a soccer victory.

I got up only once to urinate? Was that an effect of the *Ambrosia*?

Next day was like the day before, though I noted the cancer seemed a little smaller, and it did not produce the fluid it had been oozing.

Already? Four days instead of two weeks?

Next day, a friend came to see the town. She noted that the cancer seemed a lot less than three weeks ago, when I visited her in David. We drank a bit much.

I did not get up all night. I slept almost six hours.

Next two days were normal. My urine stream was stronger. I didn't have to get up during the night. The cancer was now half the size it was when I started the medicine. The eczema I have had for years was gone! I noticed that for the first time!

Eighth day, the cancer was just a bump with a scab, but there was a small bit of fluid. I used the second bag of *Ambrosia* the same way as the first.

Next two weeks were same. The cancer was now

a small hard lump, hardly noticeable. The eczema was gone. The cystocercosis ? was reduced to a very few lesions, but they were increasing. (I have used a number of things on them that seemed to be doing the job for awhile, then they came back. Same this time. Bummer!)

I noticed a slow increase in the cystocercosis, so repeated the dosage. The parasite is known to rapidly become resistant to almost anything. It stopped the increase and the lesions are less and less. I will buy some more Altamisa next time I'm in David.

It is quite simple I grow it, so simply cut off what I will need, put it in the blender with the milk, blend, and use.

For storage and later use, particularly by others, I dry the leaves and stems until a stage where they feel right (I can't explain, other than to say they become crisp.)

I then remove the larger stems and place the leaves and smaller stems into the blender and chop until powder is formed. I strain the blended material to have table salt sized and smaller pieces, which I measure and seal in plastic small bags in schedule sized packets (2 liquid ounce – 1/4 cup volume) and place them in a darker place. They can be stored at least a year this way.

If you buy the dried plant, you can simply chop and measure it for your own use.

It is not difficult or complicated, but can become tedious if you are working with much of it.

Do not mix protocols as some can nullify each other. If anything is changed, it may not work. If you mix or try other things, please inform me of the results. I am well-aware that improvements can be possible, though we have found nothing that results in improvement at this point.

In every case to this date (9/10/22) all cases where we had observation and control and that were following the protocol exactly have been successful, though slower with certain skin cancers.

I will write this with times noted. The intervals are critical, though the exact hours are solely for determing the intervals. Only in the case of use for vision correction does the time of day appear to be of importance.

We recommend starting the protocol in the afternoon, as the process seems more apt to give desired results when initiated then.

Basically, it is a matter of everything at 4 hour periods. That appears optimum for absorption and distribution in the body. 4 hours seems to be the time the higher levels of materials remain in the bloodstream.

It is the interval that is important, not the hours as listed.

A dose is ½ liquid ounce lightly packed Ambrosia in 1 cup whole milk. Mix thoroughly and swallow quickly, as the taste is not pleasant.

I find it easiest to mix the milk and material in a one cup soda bottle where I can shake it before each swallow.

```
6:00 AM    - take the iron supplement tablet
10:00 AM  - take the first dose
2:00 PM    - take the second dose
6:00 PM    - take the third dose
10:00 PM  - take the final dose
```

That's it! If you feel it necessary, you can repeat in 8 days. Thus far, that has happened only with certain skin cancers.

I have noticed several other things. I cannot say they are directly related to the *Ambrosia* treatments, but have no other change in my diet or lifestyle to explain them.

First, the nail fungus in my toenails had stopped. Most of the distorted and black nails have grown out.

Second, three days ago I was working with the computer, writing the final Clint Faraday mystery, and saw my reading glasses laying beside the mouse board. I had been working for more than three hours without my glasses? I can't see that close without the glasses! I've had to use them for more than fifteen years!

I picked up the sheet of printed research for the mystery, and read it easily. That would have been impossible a week ago!

The glasses were under the card reader. I haven't used it since the day before yesterday. I have been working without my glasses for at least three days now – and didn't know it.

The student living here said my eyes were different. They used to be a sort of muddy bluish yellow. They were now clear hazel, bluish in some light, brownish yellow in other, and sometimes a pale green.

I used to be in rock music. I play rhythm guitar and sing. Some songs would cause a coughing fit.

House of the Rising Sun (Eric Burden) the worst. No such anymore. I can do the raspy screaming stuff with no irritation.

I, in other words, had developed throat polyps. I do not know if they're gone or just arrested. They are considered pre-cancerous. I think perhaps the *Ambrosia* cancer cure works on various others. I just looked up polyps and *Artemisia* and found that it was known to reduce or cure polyps in the colon, in several studies.

I don't want to sound like those fanatic blogs. I have studied genetics, and know that what works for one person will not necessarily work for another, particularly where things not covered in the original research are concerned. The nail fungus and eyes and such may or may not work, but there is enough other information out there that all this is is corroboration. Any cure comes under those same caveats: because it worked for A & B does not mean it will work for C.

I think this protocol will work for a great majority of people. The research shows over 87% of cases, it did work. It relieved those it did not cure.

It is well worth a shot for anyone with symptoms.

It is a thing you can do yourself for less than $20 that a doctor and hospital would cost hundreds if not thousands of dollars, or the quacks, who would cost you your life's savings.

I plan to plant *Ambrosia peruviana* and try to

provide it free, or as cheaply as possible, to sufferers of Leishmaniasis here, as well as for whatever else it cures, particularly among the Indigenos, who have no money. Their culture does not require money.

Would that ours didn't.

It has been eight years since I started this. We have used it on a number of people, and have learned some things.

First, there is no overdose. I used it at 8X the strength and 2X the dosage. I noted a slight vertigo for about 4 or 5 minutes the second day. No other noticeable effects.

We have treated many types of cancer. We have had excellent results, when used as suggested.

Of those where we have been present, 47 of 47 cases were, so far as we can say at this point, cured. There has been no remission, though 4 - 5 years is not enough to define it clearly.

The only ones where we have reports that it did not work were with people, one a man who works with epoxy resin and fibreglass, finally admitted that he didn't bother with the iron, because his doctor told him to never take iron supplements if you have cancer, because the cancer absorbs and stores iron.

(Since this was first published I have researched ferrotopsis and have learned the absolute necessity of using the supplment.)
DUH! That's why it's required!
I suggested we make a fiberglass canoe! He would place the fabric on the mold, and I would apply the epoxy resin!
I heard methyl-ethyl-ketone peroxide is very

dangerous to work with, and there was only a tiny bit used, anyhow! I would just leave it out!

He looked at me as if he thought I was crazy.

We'll come next month to see if it was hardened and ready to use!

He said the resin would be a sticky, runny mess on the floor. Resin doesn't harden without the methyl-ethyl!

I looked at him. Just stared.

He suddenly slapped his head. "So the iron is the catalyst, and I'm an idiot!"

We are good friends, now. He took the cure again, and his prostate cancer is gone.

A woman who took it, with a little improvement, but no stopping the progress completely, took three dosages at eight day intervals. She said it made her feel very good, and the chemo side-effects were gone, but the cancer was still spreading.

I took her through the process with the fourth try. She did everything exactly, until blending the *Ambrosia* in milk.

"Oh, I can't do that. I'm lactose intolerant."

I explained that it was the butterfat that carried the medicinal parts into the body. Water, which she was using, did not dissolve the active parts.

We slightly warmed the water until a pat of butter [*not* margarine} would slowly melt, as it seems to carry the active ingredients through the body without allowing them to enter the cancer cell], and blended it.

She said that, at least, it tasted better!

Her breast cancer [that was spreading into her throat] was stopped within 4 days, and has shrunken to tiny hard nodules that will slowly disappear since. The throat mets were gone.

A friend is concerned with breast cancer. I believe his mother died from it. He has treated several, and with complete success. The latest two were sisters, one with a large tumor, and the other with 17 [*not a typo!*] small tumors, only one of which was more than lentil-sized. In a month, the large tumor is less than 1/5 of its volume, and is shrinking. Only the larger tumor is detectable on the sister, and it is almost gone.

The most spectacular case was a man from Germany who had liver cancer, complicated by cirrhosis. His doctors predicted he would die within four days. He was in a semi-coma, and my friend almost force-fed him the dosages.

The second day, he had diarrhea, but was able to go to the baño in the room. The third day, he walked to the front desk and sat on the porch. He felt better than he could ever remember feeling.

A week later he was walking around David. Two weeks later he flew back to Germany.

His doctors were amazed, but said you could expect a spontaneous remission, if rarely.

I asked if any of his other spontaneous remissions also remissed from cirrhosis, at the same time.

Funny. He called me a quack and stormed out,

and didn't even bother to answer me! How rude!

With leukemia, it works very quickly. You do not need the iron, because the blood carries that in ample quantity. The problem is that leukemia will come back in six or eight months, in most cases.

Luana took it, her hair grew back, she was soon playing with the other kids [9 years old] and doing quite well. It came back in a little more than 7 months – so she took it again. It has been 8 months and a week, and it hasn't reappeared. She says, if it comes back, she will just take more.

A woman who works for my friend who is doing the breast cancer study has asthma so bad she couldn't be in the same room where someone took even one small puff from a cigarette. She was constantly choking.

There was nothing to lose, so he gave her a dose.

It has been almost a year. She has not had one attack in that time.

We have one case of dengue. It cleared up in four days. We can't say it was from the *Ambrosia*, but it certainly can't hurt!

The first couple of uses will amaze you in how quickly it clears up complection problems. I am trying to find a way to stabilize the effects. I find that guava leaf extract topically and the *Amb. peruviana* internally is quite effective.

I grow various "weeds" for the research. My concentration is on *Ambrosia peruviana*, but other things come along, from time to time, that deserve attention. Most of these things have reputations of curing or relieving many illnesses. Those we haven't directly observed will not be listed here.

Before using any of these things, determine that you have no allergy to them. That is simple common sense. We all have our own reactions, programmed into our genetic matrix, that can make a boon to someone else a danger to us. Peanuts? I love them! They killed a cousin a few years back.

I will leave *Cannabis* to others, as to intense study. Our research is definitely limited.

For instance, it is limited by the difficulty in obtaining it here, and the locally grown is blah. We do find, from other credible sources, that it is effective over a broad range of problems. It's effectiveness against brain cancer is demonstrated by no less than Jimmy Carter.

Seizures of most types are controlled effectively. Certain cancers, particularly of the brain, are treated most effectively.

There is a lot of exaggeration with most things. Much good research is lost when a person becomes a fanatic. It does *not* cure all the things attributed to it. *Nothing* cures everything, but death. I am perfectly aware that *Ambrosia* is not a cure-all, but it is a cure for some things.

We have had a huge percentage of success. That will not continue forever. Our hope is to establish which of the things being tested do have these high rates of success.

Cinnamon: first, distinguish between true cinnamon and the cassia being sold as cinnamon. It tastes and smells like cinnamon, but has *none* of the medicinal reactions.
Cinnamon will often relieve type 2 diabetes greatly. It fights even the most resistant fungal infections.
Dosage: ½ teaspoon cinnamon in 1 cup water, as tea.

Guanabana: [Soursop] is very good as a preventative of many types of cancer. [and is delicious! I love guanabana chicha and ice cream!]
Dosage: I make chicha. I pint milk, a tblsp. sugar, guanabana, in blender. Serve cold.

Ginger: is excellent for internal discomforts, such as motion sickness and seasickness. A small amount of ginger in a tea or powdered will stop such distresses. It has some value as a preventative of cancer.

Coconut oil: there is nothing we've found that will cleanse the circulatory system nearly as well as coconut oil.
It will make hair grow
It dissolves cholesterol deposits in the veins and arteries and removes blockages that can cause

stroke and worse. It will clean varicose veins.

A woman who works for a friend had a clot on her lower leg that her doctor had her terrified would mean amputation if removal by laser didn't work. She took coconut oil orally and dissolved the clot in less than a week.

Take it orally, an ounce or so at a time. It has a rather unpleasant taste, but that is unimportant compared to the good it does.

Turmeric: Curcumin is perhaps the best preventative for tumors of many of the types we've encountered. It can stop the growth of some cancers. Always remember that, as with *Ambrosia peruviana* and iron, to use black pepper [piperine] with curcuma. Also use a fat source.

I use it with any curry. It is basic spice in curry. Simply put about a tblspn in spaghetti sauce or in curried dishes. Be sure to add a bit of black pepper.

Coconut oil: there is nothing we've found that will cleanse the circulatory system nearly as well as coconut oil.

It will make hair grow

It dissolves cholesterol deposits in the veins and arteries and removes blockages that can cause stroke and worse. It will clean varicose veins.

A woman who works for a friend had a clot on her lower leg that her doctor had her terrified would mean amputation if removal by laser didn't work. She took coconut oil orally and dissolved the clot in less than a week.

Take it orally, an ounce or so at a time. It has a rather unpleasant taste, but that is unimportant compared to the good it does.

New information about HIV indicates that the *Ambrosia peruviana* will relieve major symptoms and can prevent contagion. This is unconfirmed, and purely anecdotal. Research on this issue is vital.

I hope this will prove of value to many who can benefit from the information. I hope it will not be censored by a random process that does not apply.

I will appreciate any who use the protocol sending information of the results, positive or negative, to us at Facebook page: Ambrosia peruviana for cancer. Please include whether the protocol was followed exactly or if any changes whatever were made.

C. D. Moulton's works are available on most major outlets as printed or e-books. CD writes the CD Grimes, PI, mysteries, the Det. Lt. Nick Storie mysteries, the Clint Faraday mysteries, the Flight of the Maita science fiction series, books on orchid culture and many others of many types. Mystery, adventure, intrigue, science fiction, humor, fantasy, paranormal, mild erotica, and factual.

www.ingramcontent.com/pod-product-compliance
Lightning Source LLC
Chambersburg PA
CBHW052227150726
48002CB00003B/1313